10 SIMPLE HABITS

FOR

RAISING HEALTHY KIDS

HOW TO SET YOUR CHILDREN UP FOR A LONG
AND HAPPY LIFE

SERGEY YOUNG

10 SIMPLE HABITS FOR RAISING HEALTHY KIDS:
How to set your children up for a long and happy life.

In addition to the paperback edition, this book is available as an eBook and in the Adobe PDF format.

CONTENTS

Healthy and unhealthy habits start forming before kids can label them as such

CHAPTER 1

INTRODUCTION

Every parent, including me, wants their kids' lives to exceed their own when it comes to being healthy, happy, and loved. While we can't guarantee our children will grow up to live their best possible lives, it's our job as parents to do everything we can to put them on the right path. A long list of factors will impact the quality of your kids' lives, but even having the best of relationships or a well-paying dream job is arguably irrelevant without good health. Health underpins everything else—and healthy (or unhealthy) habits start forming before kids can label them as such. That's why, in my opinion, every mom or pop should prioritize teaching their children how to be healthy.

Parenting is demanding to say the least, though. I have four kids, so I'm speaking from experience here. It can be challenging to think about long-term health in the face of your kids' immediate wants and needs. And sometimes, it can be tempting to make choices that are easier in the short-term but will harm your family's health long-term. This is especially true nowadays, as there's a seemingly endless list of unhealthy but convenient options right at our fingertips—options that children often beg for! Candies, sugary drinks, fast food, and processed food can seemingly be found on every corner.

The sheer number of unhealthy options is just another reason why it's so crucial for parents to prioritize heath. Your children need to know how to make the right choices as they gradually gain their desired independence. I started parenting with an eye towards health and longevity after I was faced with my own health crisis—one that completely changed my lifestyle and diet. With this book, it's my hope that other parents won't have to wait for a similar wake-up call.

When I talk about long-term health, I don't just mean five or ten years down the line, either. Instead, I'm talking about setting your children up for health and longevity, which refers to both how long they will live and what kind of quality their life will have. Technically, longevity refers to the average lifespan of the population. But in this book, we are not just talking about the length of someone's life, but their ability to remain physically and mentally healthy during those extra years on earth.

Currently, the average life expectancy of an American is just shy of 80 years, while the number of people 90 or older has tripled in the last three decades. Those numbers are only going to expand for future generations, your children included, thanks to tremendous technological innovation. Your goal as a parent should be to help your kids make healthy choices now and as an adult, in turn allowing them to live long enough to see promising longevity technologies become mainstream.

By the time your kids are grown, our healthcare system will be fundamentally transformed, with a growing list of new technologies dramatically altering our ability to detect and handle disease. In our kids' lifetimes, too, there's a good chance life extension will be possible thanks to technology like gene editing, age-reversing drugs, stem cells, and replaceable body parts. Until then, you should be teaching your kids how to be healthy in a holistic sense—from what they eat to how many hours they sleep to how they cope with stress. One might even argue that the healthy habits I will talk about in the chapters ahead will continue to be essential or potentially even more important in the future, even if technology is more powerful to support longevity.

Indeed, setting your kids up for healthy longevity doesn't mean talking to them about living to 100 when they're a mere fraction of that age, nor does it mean explaining technological breakthroughs. Instead, it's about instilling healthy habits at an early age and reinforcing them as your children grow.

This will not be easy, of course. Mothers and fathers often struggle to tackle everyday challenges, from school to sleep. And each individual parent's ability to face these challenges will undoubtedly be affected by things outside their control—whether it's having to overcome a disability while maintaining a healthy household or just the unfortunate reality of economic inequality. Put simply, it can be hard for many parents to even afford the foods it takes to maintain a healthy diet. Being a parent isn't always a level playing field. Still, successful parenting means not only weathering these storms, but expanding ones approach and preparing your children for the future. Once again, this will ensure your children enter adulthood with a strong baseline of health for their mind, body, and soul—which in turn will allow them to live long enough to see new technologies come to fruition.

By starting young, too, there will be far less damage to undo. Every parent wants their kids to be healthy when they are adults, if not parents or grandparents, themselves. That will only happen by thinking about health and the future and longevity now.

Making healthy habits a part of your family's life and routine will set your kids up for success

THE PRINCIPLES OF LONGEVITY

This book probably isn't what you think it is. I'm not here to offer a specific diet, checklist, or prescription to you and your kids. Instead, I'm going to offer a new paradigm or perspective on health. I'm not going to insist on strict rules that must never be broken either. Instead, I'm going to define the mindset and guiding principles that will help you lead by example and guide your boys and girls down a healthy path. You don't need to memorize particular dos or don'ts. You just need to make health and longevity the guiding light for daily decisions around diet, sleep, exercise, and other things that are integral to health.

In my opinion, it's important for us to start thinking about longevity and healthspan as early as possible. This means more time for healthy decisions to turn into healthy habits—to become the default. And it's especially crucial as kids have both greater independence and greater access to information than ever before. In the past, parents were far more of an information filter for their kids. Now, children are faced with social media, advertising, and news from all directions at a far younger age, which often lead them towards unhealthy habits and decisions. It's very difficult for parents to be the primary filter for their kids these days, so we need to prepare them to make smart, healthy decisions on their own.

Making healthy habits a part of your family's life and routine—from minimizing processed foods to engaging in sufficient daily activity—will set your kids up for success. With the help of this book, you can put your children squarely on the path to 100. Of course, other adults come into contact with your children as well. Lots of people, from grandparents to teachers, try to use sweets as a gift or reward. As a parent, part of your role is to create a healthy longevity bubble around your children. While you can't control every variable, you can engage in conversations with relatives, friends' parents, and schools in an attempt to push those people towards healthier choices as well.

This might sound serious and a bit daunting, but we should approach longevity playfully. You can have fun while being healthy, and you can occasionally ignore many of the suggestions I'm going to outline in this book. Nobody is perfect. Every July, for instance, I take my younger kids to McDonald's (yes, once a year!). And sometimes, we enjoy other cheat meals together. This reminds us not to take things too seriously and to simply enjoy ourselves sometimes! But overall, my wife, kids and I have reached a very healthy baseline with regard to everything from eating to stress management. In this book, I'll share with you how to do the same.

WHO IS SERGEY YOUNG?

I know how difficult it can be to make sense of all the information that exists about health and longevity, much less to put it into practice. Trust me—I've been studying this stuff for years! I also understand that getting your kids to follow your guidance is a whole different ball game. I have four kids myself, though one is already grown: Nikita is 22, Timothy is 10, Polina is 7, and Max is 3. With each comes a different parenting challenge.

While your kids may have one idea of what will improve their lives — likely a new toy or sweet snack — it's your job as a parent to think longer term. Of course, I couldn't think long term about my kids' health until I was doing it for myself. For me, the first step was understanding what a healthy life looked like, so I could both model the right behavior and teach the right habits. I didn't really think too much about health until six years ago. I had high cholesterol level, which caused a doctor to tell me I'd have to take a pill every day for the rest of my life. That prospect wasn't appealing to me, so I started doing my own research. As I did, I realized how common it is for people to be struggling with health—which means they're struggling to set their kids up for success too.

Fast forward a few years and what started as a journey to figure out how I could lower my cholesterol without taking a statin has morphed into a career. I've been an investor for over 20 years. As I learned more about health and longevity, starting a fund focused on companies in the space was a natural next step. Since launching that fund, I've spent years learning from everyone I could—academics, investors, and innovators from Boston, the biotech capital of the world, to Silicon Valley, the tech capital of the world—about how we can all live longer.

I also co-lead an upcoming nonprofit age reversal tech competition (an XPRIZE initiative) and have helped 300,000 employees at various organizations around the globe improve their health through a free program called "Longevity at Work." I've seen what works with regard to health and healthspan — and what doesn't.

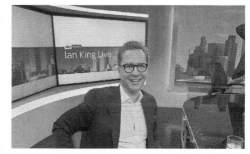

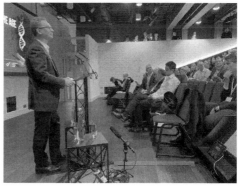

These experiences have also helped me be a better parent, especially when it comes to preparing my children to live long, healthy lives. The goal of this book is to take all the facts and secrets about longevity that I've learned, especially as it pertains to parenting, and share it with you in a quick, digestible format. Once again, this book isn't about checklists or rules. It's about having the right overarching health paradigm to guide you and your family's health choices—today, tomorrow, and on your kid's 100th birthday. Still, I will break my advice into buckets so it's easy to follow.

Before we dig into details I want to thank Claudio Gienal, Lana Asprey, Dr. Ildiko Edenhoffer for sharing their personal stories and providing professional advice and feedback on the content of this book.

WHAT TO EXPECT

Now that I've explained the philosophy behind this book, it's time to get into the action. I've broken the book into 10 chapters for you, each focusing on one component of longevity and how it relates to kids.

In **Chapter 1**, I'll share how to teach boys and girls about **healthy eating**. In **Chapter 2**, we'll talk about the importance of **drinking water**. In **Chapter 3**, I'll tell you how to approach **doctor's visits**. In **Chapter 4**, we'll tackle the importance of **daily activity and movement**.

We'll cover the importance of **sleep** in **Chapter 5** and the balanced use of **gadgets** in **Chapter 6**. **Chapter 7** will focus on **the ability to relax and meditate**, followed by the importance of **kindness and gratitude** in **Chapter 8**. Finally, we'll talk about the importance of **being social** in **Chapter 9** and **overall safety** in **Chapter 10**.

This is all very exciting and transformative. Let's get started!

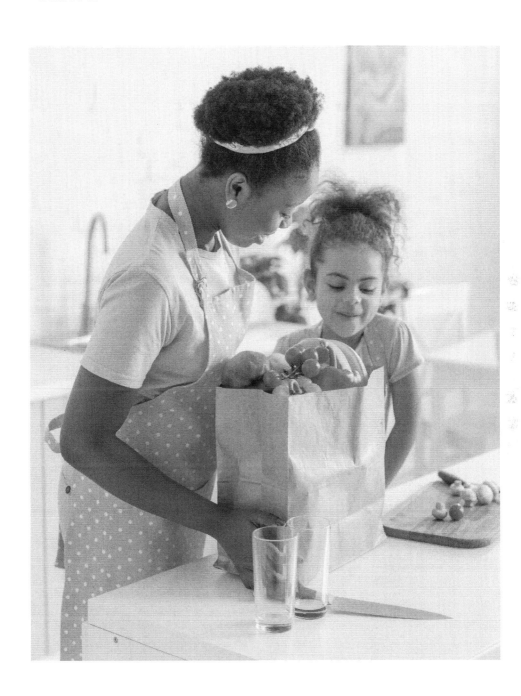

CHAPTER 2

YOU ARE WHAT YOU EAT

When it comes to making choices today that will ensure your family's health and happiness tomorrow, perhaps nothing is more powerful than food. You might think of meals as family time or social time or maybe just additional items on your to-do list, but they're also the cornerstone of longevity. I talk in more detail about the importance of food for health and longevity in my previous book, "10 Simple Principles of a Healthy Diet: Buy the book here: www.sergeyyoung.com/10principles How to Lose Weight, Look Young, and Live Longer". Many common health problems that adults encounter—such as high blood pressure, heart disease, diabetes, and more—have poor food choices at their root. Meanwhile, healthier choices offer healing, detoxification, and even anti-aging effects. It's very easy for me to guess which of those two options you prefer for your children.

Unfortunately, most American children have unhealthy habits. Researchers at Tufts University looked at the diets of 31,000 American kids (aged 2 to 19) across the country and found that 56% had diets of poor nutritional quality. Relatedly, childhood obesity in the U.S. is a growing problem; its prevalence has doubled in children and tripled in teens during the past 30 years. According to a study in the New England Journal of Medicine, this uptrend could shorten life spans by as much as five years. Young adults who are overweight have a 70% chance of being overweight when they grow up, while half of all American adults are projected to be obese by 2030. Obesity is linked to 13 types of cancer, type-2 diabetes, heart disease, and more.

You probably already know that it's important for kids to eat well—and you probably know why. It doesn't just affect their physical health, but also their mental health, energy, and focus. As a study published by The American Health Association in 2014 put it: "a poor quality diet that is lacking nutrient-dense foods may lead to nutrient deficiencies that have been associated with mental health issues." Further solidifying the notion that diet has direct ties to mental health. Plus, healthy meals throughout childhood can create crucial habits that will hopefully extend into adulthood—and thus extend your kids' healthy lives.

Explain to boys and girls—on an ongoing basis and in entertaining ways—that what they eat is connected to their physical health, growth, strength, performance at school, and ability to have fun with friends

The challenging part, of course, is getting your kids to actually eat the green beans you put on their plate and getting them to seek out greens in general when they're one day making food choices of their own. The aforementioned research out of Tufts University found that teenagers had the worst diets of all! So the question, really, is how: how can parents get their kids to understand the importance of nutrition and more or less default to healthy choices?

The first step is education. Without the right knowledge, it's far harder to make the right choices. You don't need to share scary statistics with your 12-year-old, though. Instead, explain to boys and girls—on an ongoing basis and in entertaining ways—that what they eat is connected to their physical health, growth, strength, performance at school, and ability to have fun with friends. You can also add that it will prevent future diseases that could impact their ability to do things they enjoy.

A lot of your kids' food education should be far more subtle, though. By cooking together, going to the farmer's market, and discussing food on an ongoing basis, you'll be laying a strong foundation for your children. Remember, your goal as a parent should be to help your kids make the right food choices now and as an adult to ensure they live long enough to see promising life extension technologies become more accessible and affordable.

A gentle and effective food education can come by simply making it fun to shop for, cook, and eat healthy foods. When it comes to instilling healthy and sustainable food habits, don't just focus on all the things your kids can't have! Instead, engage with a wide range of healthy foods in your family's day-to-day life and try to spark your kids' curiosity whenever possible.

I call walnuts "brain nuts," for example, because they look like a brain and feed our brains! I tell my kids they will help them get smarter faster. Additionally, my children know that carrots are good for their eyes while fermented foods are good for their tummy. When they don't want to eat certain food, I say it's not for them, but for their tiny microorganisms, which fight viruses and bad bacteria on their behalf.

We also buy a lot of whole foods—including some my children are less familiar with—and see if they know where it grows, what it's usually served with, or why it's good for them. If they don't know a particular food, we look it up together. Cooking together is a great way to educate your children as well, as it also allows you and your kids to explore different cultures, flavors, and cooking styles! Plus, it's always nice to have a helper in the kitchen!

If you're not a chef yourself, that's okay. There are plenty of fun and simple cooking classes available these days. Additionally, growing a garden (even a small one by a window or outside), making regular trips to the farmer's market, or taking a one-off trip to a local farm are all great ways to get your children acquainted with the greens and veggies that should make up the bulk of their diet.

The farmer's market is my personal favorite because it's a great weekend family trip. Give your kid a basket and a budget, and let them pick stuff out! Challenge them to find foods that match all the colors of the rainbow and quiz them on food names. Pretty soon, your kids will be waking you up on the weekends as if it's Christmas morning—begging you to take them to buy some fresh veggies!

Actress Kristen Bell educates her children in many of the ways I'm suggesting here. As she put it: "They are interested in the fact that I care so much about food. [We] talk about a colorful plate when I'm cutting up vegetables for a platter or a dish. We talk about what goes into it and why it's good for your body."

This quote alludes to another key part of your kids' nutritional education: leading by example. When your children are young, you have the most control over what goes on their plates. But they're also learning from what you put on your own plate. If there's one easy shortcut to healthy eating, it's emphasizing balanced diet based on whole plants. For those of us who grew up with a food pyramid guiding our choices, think of fruits and vegetables as the base.

If you want your kids to eat certain foods, you should be eating them too! So be sure to take every opportunity to spread that healthy rainbow of vegetables across each meal you prepare, and enjoy its benefits to your own life! Going to the farmer's market is also a great bet because it ensures you and your kids are eating foods that are local, seasonal, and organic as opposed to imported, out-of-season, and conventionally grown. Similarly, if you consume animal product, make sure you're opting for organic meat and poultry and organic wild fish. Gwyneth Paltrow, for instance, cooks for her children every night. She feeds them organic foods, while avoiding heavily processed or genetically modified ones.

Along the same lines, it's crucial to clear your fridge and pantry of all those tempting, unhealthy snacks. By simply dumping the bad stuff and keeping dangerous or unhealthy foods totally out of reach, you've solved 80% of the problem. It's far easier to create good habits when good food choices are right at your fingertips and bad ones aren't teasing you every second of the day! Processed foods are made to keep you coming back for more. They add about 500 calories per day to your diet, and excess calories have been shown to shorten lifespans.

Plus, many of them seem relatively harmless. But sweetened or flavored yogurt, cereal, granola bars, and lots of flavored drinks are packed with sugar. As Professor Juliana Cohen put it: "Sugar in small doses is okay, but with the portion sizes most people are used to today, we've lost perspective on moderation." The American Heart Association recommends no more than 100 calories from added sugar a day for children older than age 2. That translates to about 24 grams. For comparison, a 12-ounce can of Coca-Cola contains 39 grams—more than the daily limit! When it comes to keeping sugary and processed foods away from your kids, the phrase "out of sight, out of mind" is a helpful one to live by.

The good news is that you don't have to worry about reading labels and counting calories or grams of sugar if you stick to fresh, whole, organic foods. And you should make those options available to your children as much as possible. Have them eat breakfast at home before school and send them off with healthy snacks like veggies and nuts. This way they can avoid being concerned with other more tempting options while they're out of the house. Make a bowl of fruits always accessible in the kitchen, so your kids can snack whenever they want. Also, talk to grandparents, friends' parents, and teachers about the habits you are trying to reinforce—and why.

Last but not least, when it comes to cooking your own food, don't skip dessert! My kids eat regular candy here and there, but we usually opt for spinning up a frozen smoothie or making our own chocolate. It's more fun anyway because you get to play with your dessert before you eat it. Similarly, make rituals and rewards center on good, nutritious food as well. If you do buy cakes, keep in mind that those sold in stores often have preservatives, trans fats, and unnatural additives for color and smell. Opting for homemade cakes, cupcakes, and pies, or purchasing them from small family-owned bakeries or freelance pastry-chefs is better.

All in all, if you educate your kids, expose them to healthy foods, and lead by example, you're off to a great start. Eating and cooking together doesn't just represent the foundation of your kids' long-term health. It can be fun too!

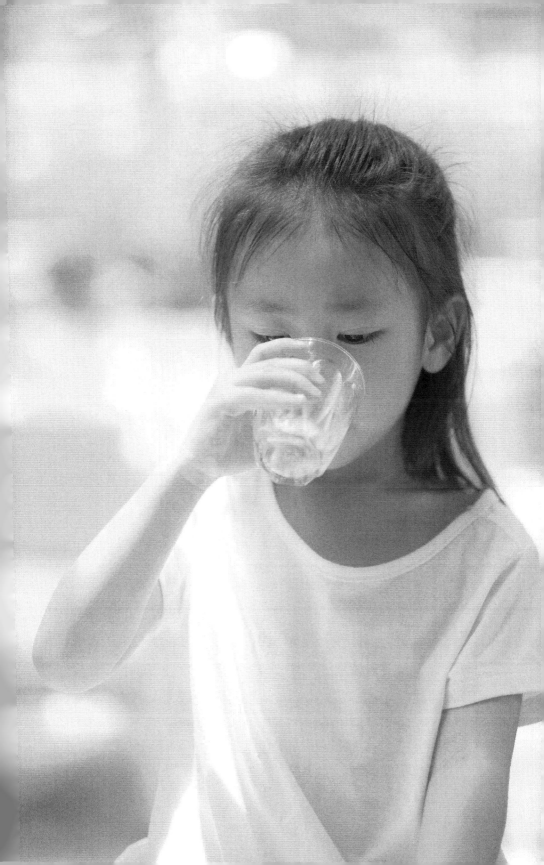

CHAPTER 3

FALL IN LOVE WITH WATER!

We all know that health is multifaceted and complex. While diet is indeed the foundation of a long, healthy, happy life, it doesn't stop there. The most related component of health is what your kids are drinking, particularly because there's often a tremendous amount of sugar hiding in their cups. The best way to avoid that sugar is relatively simple: teach them to reach for water. This will ensure they are hydrated and healthy, instilling good habits that will stay with them for life.

There's a good chance you know that sugar wreaks havoc on health. But just in case, let's run through the basics. Even if juice has fruit in the name, that "fruit" has been stripped of all the fiber that makes it good for you. And in most cases, they've replaced that fiber with high amounts of processed sugars.

A 2018 Purdue University study found that sugary beverages (fruit juice, soda, and sports drinks) are the greatest source of sugar in the average kid's diet. Drinking juice can often lead kids to crave sugar more broadly too. And some doctors suggest children under 2 should have no added sugar at all.

One cup of freshly squeezed orange juice has 21 grams of sugar—the same amount you'd get from eating 2.5 oranges. Eating the actual oranges is a better option. It takes longer so the sugar absorption is slower, which is better for your body.

Research done on flies showed that a high-sugar diet shortened their lifespans by 7 percent, even if the diet later improved. A study published in a journal called Nutrition found that kids who consumed sugary drinks tended to weigh more than kids who did not—and we already covered the risks that accompany obesity. When the children being studied replaced those sugary drinks with milk or water, body weight dropped. On top of that, sugary drinks increase the risks of cardiovascular disease and the chance of death from all causes.

Research has also shown a sudden rise in kidney stones amongst teens and adolescents over the last 15 years. According to The Children's Hospital of Philadelphia, the prevalence of kidney stones has nearly doubled, leading the Children's Hospital to begin conducting a PUSH study in 2017 (PUSH standing for "Prevention of Urinary Stones with Hydration") hoping to map the correlation between the formation of stones and poor hydration habits.

Again, these statistics are to convince you of the importance of water—not for you to scare your kids! Getting your kids to drink water is important both so they avoid drinks with more sugar and calories, and also because hydration itself is crucial to health. Besides, drinking water is cheaper than buying soda and juice too!

If your kids don't love water, explain to them how much their bodies rely on it! Children are three-quarters water, as are their brains specifically. Additionally, their lungs are 90% water and their blood is 85% water. Everyone needs water so our blood can carry oxygen to our cells, so our bodies can fight off illness, so we can digest our food, and so we can regulate our temperatures. And that's just a quick sample of all the things water helps our bodies do.

Most of us don't know how much water kids should drink to stay properly hydrated. According to the American Academy of Pediatrics, to stay well hydrated, children ages 1-3 years need ~ 4 cups of non-sugary beverages per day, including water. 4-8 year olds need around 5 cups, and older children 7-8 cups per day. These amounts vary by individual and may need to be adjusted.

"

Getting your kids to drink more water is, much like getting them to eat more veggies, all about making it fun

Some signs that your children may not be drinking enough water are dark urine, constipation, headaches, a lack of concentration, or cracked lips. You don't need to measure every cup of water that your kids consume, though. Just keep an eye on these signs, eliminate sugary drinks, and encourage as much water consumption as possible—especially if your kids are extremely active, sick, or spending a lot of time in the heat.

Getting your kids to drink more water is, much like getting them to eat more veggies, all about making it fun. In fact, the more of these tips you can turn into fun games, the better.

Let your girl or boy pick out a fun water bottle that you can pack when they head to school. You could make an afternoon out of buying a new water bottle and decorating it with colorful stickers or markers. You can then encourage them to always hold onto their water bottle by playing a game where you ask if they have their bottle at random throughout the week. If they have it by their side, reward them with a new sticker to add to their bottle. If they think water is boring, try adding fruit slices for flavor. Place a cup of water by their bed so that they can drink first thing in the morning.

Drink water with your kids too—perhaps in your own fun water bottle or in colorful glasses. Add fun ice cubes and straws, have contests to see who can drink the most water, and talk about how different you feel when you eat healthy foods and stay hydrated vs. when you opt for processed, sugary options. If you also struggle with drinking enough water, check out my previous book, "10 Simple Principles of a Healthy Diet", where I share more tips on how to get used to staying hydrated.

It's when we normalize the consumption of water, that it becomes the default. Water should be viewed as the first and regular option. When it is, sugary options like juice or soda innately become what they should be: a treat every once and a while. By making water consumption part of your family's routine—and by making it fun—your children will be used to drinking enough water and won't be craving cups of sugary fruit juice or soda. Pair that with healthy foods and you're off to a great start.

Your kids are going to have relationships with food and drink throughout their whole lives. By setting a good example and teaching them the right choices, you're putting them on the path to health, happiness and longevity—not disease.

CHAPTER 4

BEFRIEND YOUR DOCTOR

Dodging disease (and helping your kids do the same) isn't solely about diet, though. In fact, I consider healthy eating part of the first building block of longevity, which focuses on all the things we can do now to extend our lives. The second and third blocks, meanwhile, depend upon a greater degree of technological innovation and scientific breakthroughs.

The second building block in particular is important to parents. It includes technologies that are in development now or just around the corner: promising advances in disease prevention, regenerative medicine, genome therapy and editing, AI-based diagnostics and drug discovery, and smart hospitals, to name a few. Put simply, medicine is going to look very different for our kids when they're finally adults. For instance, early-diagnosis technologies, which are crucial to extending our lifespans, will most likely be normal to them.

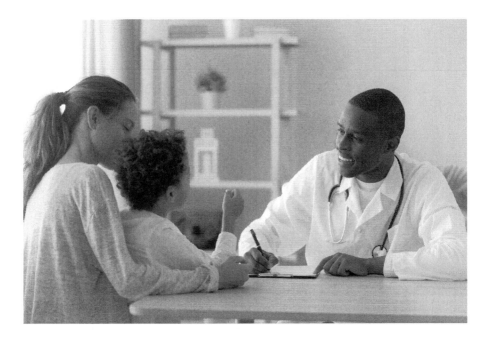

Making doctor's visits a habit will put them in a position to actually take advantage of new medical technologies as they become available

While preventing disease is the goal, catching one early is the next best option. When diseases are detected early, they are far less likely to be deadly. Advanced technologies that improve diagnostics will play a large role in your children's health as they age—but only if they're in a position to use them. Thus, in addition to teaching your children to eat right, you should also make sure they build a strong relationship with their doctor.

Making doctor's visits a habit—I recommend having your kids go at least twice a year—will put them in a position to actually take advantage of new medical technologies as they become available. At the risk of stating the obvious, it's hard to get screened for a disease if you don't visit the doctor (though technology is slowly changing that).

How exactly can technology improve diagnostics and medicine? To start, artificial intelligence (AI) is being used for everything from cancer detection to MRIs. For example, a company called Freenome uses AI to decode the body's own warning signs for cancer—biomarker patterns that were once too complex to be interpreted for a diagnosis. Additionally, Exo Imaging offers an AI-enabled handheld ultrasound device, Eko Health created an AI-enabled digital stethoscope for cardiovascular health diagnostics, and researchers at UCL have been doing cardiac MRI scans with AI. Once again, the earlier medical professionals can diagnose a problem, the better chance they have of fixing it.

Going to the doctor regularly will make it so your kids are prepared to take advantage of these technologies down the line. Plus, visiting a doctor regularly will help your children actually build a relationship and learn to trust doctors, which is just as important as care. My kids go every six months—January and July are for dental visits, while April and October are for pediatric visits—and they get a healthy treat after each one!

Of course, going to the doctor regularly comes with more immediate benefits as well. It's good to have basic checkups and bloodwork to ensure development, vision, and other aspects of your kids' health look normal. Also, the sooner boys and girls establish a baseline of what "healthy" looks like, the more effectively healthcare can be applied as time goes by.

This relates to the concept of personalized medicine, which is also part of the second building block of longevity. For some people, just knowing what genes they have can be the difference between life and death. Less than two decades ago, sequencing the whole human genome cost almost $3 billion and took more than 10 years. Today, it costs a few hundred dollars and the process takes as little as an hour. Having a large amount of information about the human genome will allow us to better assess an individual's risk for disease and target treatments accordingly.

Add it up, and there's good reason to be optimistic about our ability to fight disease and prevent premature death, especially in the decades to come. Already, countless technologies are poised to revolutionize medicine. This will be of tremendous importance to your children's health as they grow up. But for now, the main thing to do as a parent is get your kids used to going to the doctor.

While it's not reasonable to expect you can make going to the doctor as fun as going to the farmer's market, there are still plenty of ways you can reinforce a good relationship with the medical world. First, model good behavior by going regularly yourself. We can't expect our kids to value a relationship with a doctor if we don't have one ourselves. Next, try to always talk about doctors in a positive light. Sometimes the world of medicine can be a confusing and frustrating one. Nevertheless, it's important to instill a solid respect for the medical profession in our children. This means speaking well of doctors and how necessary they are to our quality of life.

Third, build positive relationships with all healthcare professionals you encounter, including your kids'. It's one thing to sing their praises, but it's another to build on that in front of your children by showing them how to foster a positive relationship with medical professionals. And last but not least, reward your kids for going to their regular doctor's visits. It can be as simple and easy as making sure your kids get a treat after a doctor's visit, or as bold and fun as taking them to the movies that same evening.

Regardless of how you choose to positively reinforce doctors visits, it's always a good idea to consistently do so.

In addition to the immediate health benefits of regular medical care, befriending your doctor will also have a long-term pay-off, as your kids will be more likely to use and benefit from numerous technologies that are just around the corner.

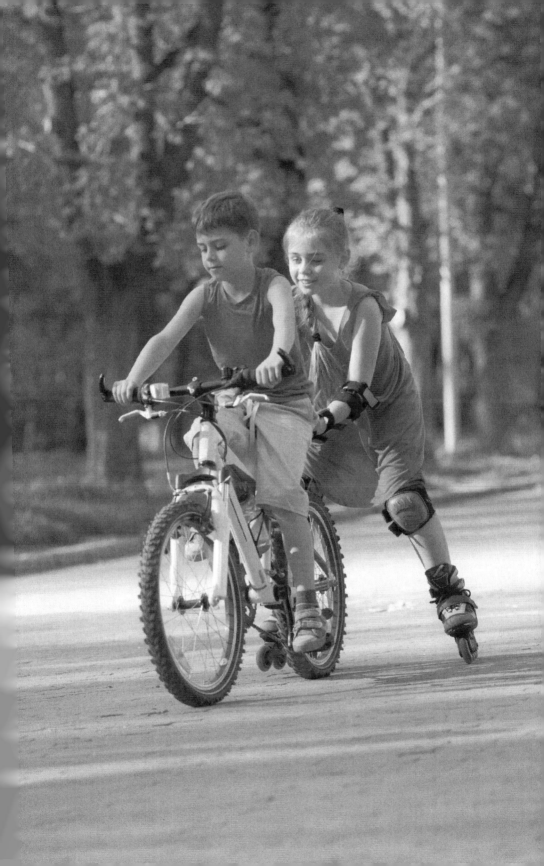

CHAPTER 5

GET MOVIN'!

While doctors can support you and your children's health, there's one thing arguably more powerful than anything a white coat can prescribe: exercise. No matter the situation, a little fresh air and movement always seems to make things better. I'm not just speculating here, either. Movement has made my family, myself included, happier and healthier. Additionally, numerous studies have documented the positive benefits that physical activity has on people's health and longevity.

According to records, organized exercise existed in ancient China as far back as 2500 BC. Fast forward to the 1950s and studies conducted in London showed that increased physical activity reduced the risk of coronary heart disease—currently the leading cause of death in the United States. More recent studies, meanwhile, have demonstrated that burning a mere 1,000 calories per week is associated with a 20% to 30% reduction in mortality.

Movement, especially when combined with the healthy eating principles outlined earlier, also lowers the risk of diabetes and cancer. As few as 15 minutes of moderate exercise per day can add up to seven years to one's life. For youth, though, at least 60 minutes per day is recommended. It's our job as moms and dads to both model an active lifestyle and nudge our kids down a similarly active path.

The easiest way to ensure your children reap the benefits of physical activity is to sign them up for sports. The key, in my opinion, is letting boys and girls try as many sports as possible. Experiment and see what sticks! If they find an activity they love—and make friends doing it—there's a far higher chance they'll continue to play as they grow. Whether it's basketball, jiu-jitsu or trampolines, the point is simply to get moving.

Stretching should also be part of a daily physical activity routine. It seems that flexibility comes naturally to children, but parents must teach kids to stretch properly. Stretching improves mobility, which is important for sports performance and injury prevention in growing children; decreases muscle stiffness and increases range of motion; reduces muscular tension and enhances muscular relaxation. Both you and your kids will enjoy these benefits if you stretch together and even more if you make it fun.

Once again, sports have physical, mental, and social benefits for children. Youth who play sports have stronger bones and muscles and are less likely to be overweight. A study of over 9,000 children found that kids who were exposed to adverse childhood experiences reported better mental health as adults when they played sports. The great thing about sports, too, is that it makes physical activity routine, as most teams provide practice and workout schedules. Plus, team sports have a social component—another key lever for health and longevity.

But sports aren't the only way you can (or should) work movement into your family's life. I'm a huge fan of walking and love to challenge my kids to take more steps than me on any given day. This is an easy activity to pair with other aspects of day-to-day life. For instance, if my children want to have a conversation with me regarding something they may want or an activity they want to try, I take them on a walk to talk about it. It's an easy way to get them out of the house and get some time away from screens and distractions, listen to them, all the while getting in some steps.

This is actually becoming more commonplace in the workplace as well. Companies are starting to hold meetings on hikes as a way to combat the sedentary nature of the modern era. We spend so much of our days sitting behind a screen, and our children are no exception. It helps to normalize walking as a common activity. Walking should be presented as a way to either take a break from the stresses of the world, or to focus on a specific thought and give it the attention it deserves.

If your children have an Apple Watch or other fitness tracker, you already have an easy way to capture their attention with regard to walking. Teach them to keep an eye on how many steps they take, how long they spend standing, and how many active calories they burn. A family competition is a great way to get everyone off the couch.

Additionally, small changes in your routine—like parking as far away as possible from the grocery store—can add up and make a big impact. A study of adults showed that walking 8,000 steps per day instead of 4,000 steps halved the mortality rate. No matter the tactic, the key is to model a lifestyle in which movement is the norm. If your children have an active baseline, they're more likely to carry good habits into adulthood.

All in all, exercise is particularly important for boys and girls—both because of its immediate benefits and its potential to shape their health down the road. One study measured the activity levels of nearly 8,000 people when they were 14 years old, then again when they were 31. The results were clear: participation in sports was associated with higher levels of physical activity later in life—which translates to better health and longevity.

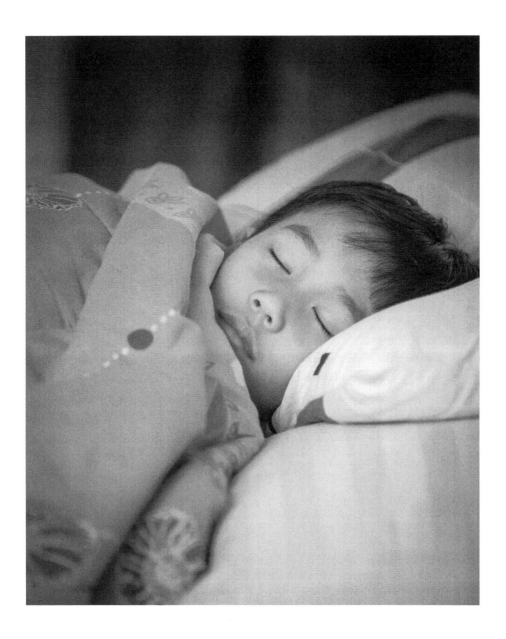

Every night when we sleep we are essentially visiting the top health clinic in the world

CHAPTER 6

PRIORITIZE REST

One thing adults tend to value more than our youthful counterparts is sleep. As a teenager, staying up late is all the rage. As adults, everyone wishes for an extra hour or two of shut-eye. It's not just because we all tend to be in better moods when we're properly rested, either. Sleep, like exercise, comes with a laundry list of health benefits. As one health expert put it, every night when we sleep we are essentially visiting the top health clinic in the world.

Unfortunately, most children don't think of sleep this way. Ask any kid and they'll most likely tell you they hate sleeping. Children tend to think it's a waste of time because they can't play or read if they're asleep. I suspect many parents reinforce a negative attitude towards sleep by using it as a punishment, too. For example, some people send their kids to bed early if they get in trouble or don't complete their chores. This is a huge mistake.

Sleep should be framed as not just a luxury, but a necessity!

While adults need an average of 8 hours of sleep per night, children need even more. Johns Hopkins suggests that children from the ages of 13 to 18 need 8 to 10 hours; those aged 6 to 12 need 9 to 12 hours; kids aged 3 to 5 need 10 to 13 hours and kids younger might need as many as 12 to 16 per day! That's a lot of rest during their most formative of years.

Meanwhile, thousands upon thousands of studies have linked getting less than 7 hours of sleep to everything from heart disease to stroke. And children who get insufficient sleep have been shown to have numerous struggles as a result, from weaker immune systems to future cardiovascular risks. Timing is also very important, for example: sleeping from 12 am until 8 am tends to allow for less deep sleep—the most restorative and rejuvenating sleep stage--then sleeping from 10 pm until 6 am for most people.

You don't have to scare your kids with fear-mongering facts, though. Instead, remind them that children need rest in order to grow—and in order to stay healthy while doing so. The bulk of growth hormones are released shortly after the start of a deep sleep. These hormones promote tissue growth that not only manifests in your children's development, but it also repairs blood vessels to promote healing. Sleep also helps our body by bolstering the production of white blood cells, which are imperative against the fight of viruses and bacteria. As is the case with healthy eating, educating your children about sleep cycles and the benefits of sleep should help them see this "activity" in a more positive light.

You can also introduce your kids to the concept of a "circadian rhythm" and why our bodies need different stages of sleep to recover different parts of our body and brain. Stress the need for consistency when it comes to sleep, not just with the amount of hours, but with regular bedtimes and a set time to wake up. Remind your children that, without sleep, they won't have the proper amount of energy to be able to do any of the things they enjoy, like playing sports or playing with friends.

Another way to positively reinforce sleep, especially as your kids get older, is to not be a stickler about nap times. Put simply, let your children nap if they want to. Sometimes, my daughter Polina likes to come to work with me. The drive home at the end of the day only takes 15 minutes and she uses it to get some shut-eye. While the United States doesn't embrace nap culture, countless other countries do. I suggest following their lead. There's no reason to push through if you're exhausted. Similarly, there's no reason to be religious about getting exactly 8 hours each night. Just remind your children of its importance and do your best to get them into a healthy routine.

Many fitness trackers allow you to tally sleep in addition to steps. The Oura Ring and Apple Watch are great ways to help your kids get interested in how they are sleeping.

Additionally, make sure your family's bedrooms are prepared for sleep. Studies show the ideal conditions for deep, restorative sleep are a cool temperature (about 65°F or 18°C) and absolute darkness. I'm a huge fan of black-out curtains for this reason. But if you're looking for something a bit different, white or pink noise has shown to reduce the onset of sleep by nearly 40% according to the Sleep Foundation. And it's been proven to especially help with infants who need help getting to bed. Not only is this approach good for setting an environment that's supportive of getting proper sleep, but it's also an extremely beneficial tool for parents who live in areas where there's a lot of competing external noise around bedtime.

Finally, having a pre-bed routine makes it easier to get the right amount of shut-eye each night. For instance, perhaps your kids shower, read, then go to sleep every evening. The more they do it, the more automatic it will be. I try to make sure to read to my children for ten minutes every evening. It truly works for me and my kids. I can always see them wind down and fall into a trance as they drift away to the sounds of a story. I think as long as you've established a consistent, structured bedtime routine, you'll be doing your children wonders with regards to their relationship to sleep, and the respect they'll grow up having for a good night's rest.

And when it comes to gadgets, make sure your children power down at least one hour before bed. As you may already know, our gadgets emit high intensity blue light that our brain perceives as daylight. When exposed to this light during the evening hours, it stops the production of melatonin that our body uses to wind down. So be sure to put away the screens before your bedtime routine even starts.

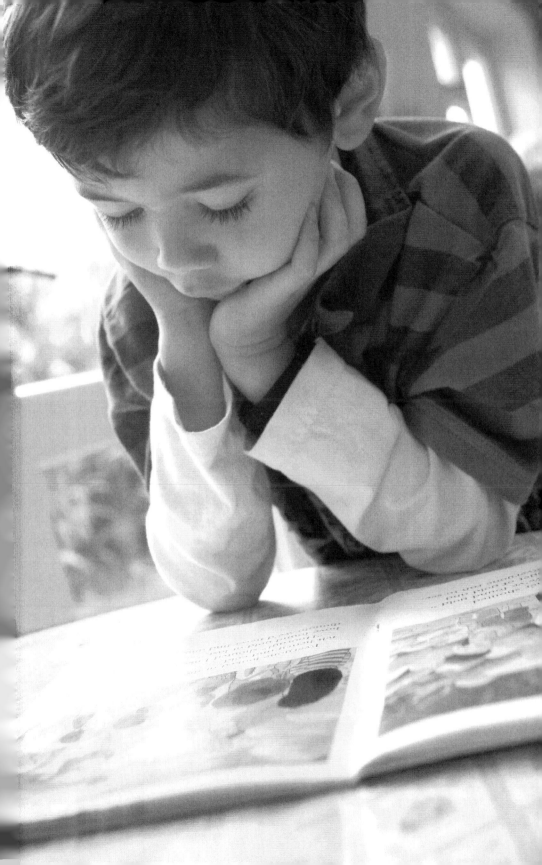

CHAPTER 7

USE GADGETS WISELY

Thus far, I've mentioned a few gadgets that are useful for teaching your children healthy habits, such as wearables that track activity and sleep. But technology is always a hot-button issue in the parenting world. Many moms and dads are rightfully concerned about the amount of time their kids spend using them.

My advice is relatively simple: use gadgets wisely. Gadgets and screens are a part of all kids' lives now, with at least some school being conducted online. Trying to fully eliminate them is a fool's errand. Instead, try to steer your kids towards gadgets that nudge healthy habits. Also, limit their screen time for entertainment.

Simply taking a kids' tablet away isn't enough to solve the problem, instead, be sure to provide fun alternatives

According to the World Health Organization, children between the ages of 2 and 4 should limit screen time to an hour per day. And when kids are older, the recommended limit is two hours. Yet on average, kids spend more than 7 hours in front of a screen for entertainment each day. This is concerning, particularly when we are talking about health and longevity. Greater screen time is associated with worse development, worse sleep, and other health issues. And time spent in front of a screen is time spent not moving.

It's hard to know the "correct" amount of time we should allow our children to watch screens. I "borrowed" a rule from my dear friend Claudio Gienal, CEO of AXA UK & Ireland, where my kids are allowed 20 minutes of daily screen time on weekdays, and one hour on weekends or holidays. This rule is consistent with the American Academy of Pediatrics recommendations stating that children younger than 18 months should not use screen media other than video-chatting; children 2 to 5 years of age should limit screen use to 1 hour per day of high-quality programming, and for children older than 6 parents and caregivers should place consistent limits on the time spent using media, and make sure media does not take the place of adequate sleep, physical activity and other behaviors essential to health.

Simply taking a kids' tablet away isn't enough to solve the problem, though. Instead, be sure to provide fun alternatives. Think up some outdoor adventures or set up an arts and crafts table somewhere in the house. You can also minimize screen time by having your kids read paper books or listen to audiobooks.

Celebrities all have different approaches to the screen time issue. Hugh Jackman only lets his kids have screen time on weekends, while Jennifer Lopez only allows it on Sundays. Chrissy Tiegan tries to enthusiastically suggest alternatives when her daughter begs for her smartphone. And Jessica Alba limits her own screen time in order to set a good example for her kids. No matter what approach you take, the point is to get your kids in the habit of entertaining themselves without technology— not to ban it completely.

As important as it is to manage the amount of time your kids spend in front of a screen, it's just as important to be involved in what they're doing when they're on their screens. Kids have an unprecedented amount of access to information this day and age.

This reality found its way into my own life once during a visit with a close friend of mine. I was being entertained by his two little daughters aged 5 and 7, and they began to tell me stories about Nike and Adidas. As anyone could imagine, I found this to be very amusing. How could these two little girls know so much about the workings and history of two huge corporations? But upon further investigation, we found that they had been listening to a podcast series. I was surprised. I mean, they knew more about these companies than I did!

But it was an eye opening moment for me with regards to just how easy it is for information to make its way to the eyes and ears of our children. Unlike the story with my friend's daughters, sometimes even seemingly harmless apps, podcasts, websites and films can sneak in a lot of information you may not feel comfortable with your kids having. Much like the issue of screen time, there's no "right answer" for how to regulate what our children find, or ingest while on their screens. I believe that communication is your most trustworthy ally when it comes to being proactive in managing your kids' relationship with their screens. Learn about their interests and then do some research on your own to find sources you can refer to your child. This not only shows your child that you're interested in learning about who they are and who they're becoming, but it gives you the opportunity to vet sources and provide them with options that make you feel more comfortable with their screen habits.

There's a lot of kid friendly apps just a click away, and remember that there's plenty of opportunities for children to not only be entertained by their screens, but to be educated as well! Verywellfamily.com recently published the best educational apps of 2021 and amongst them were apps like Quizlet, Prodigy, and Hopscotch. These are all apps dedicated to making learning fun by creating entertaining yet insightful exercises for kids.

Along with communication, definitely remember to utilize options out there like parental locks and content blockers. Apps like Bark, Net Nanny, or even just device settings are simple, useful tools at our disposal as parents. Using apps like these can really bring you some peace of mind when you can't be as tuned in to every little thing your child is doing while on their screen. But to call back to communication, be sure to take the time to discuss decisions you make regarding how you limit your kids access to the world of information at their fingertips. Your children need to understand what's out there and how easy it is to stumble across things that they're not ready to see or learn.

It's always worth opening a dialogue with other parents you and you children interact with. It's an obvious fact that different households operate differently, so it's always worth taking the time to communicate your views on screen time, and learn about other ways your friends are handling this topic. And if necessary, don't feel nervous about suggesting a shared policy on screen time. This way, you can rest assured your kids are in good hands while they're away from home, and all the parents are on the same page.

CHAPTER 8

TEACH MEDITATION

An unfortunate trend we've noticed in the U.S. and other countries is that instead of being young and carefree, children and teens are generally stressed out. According to the American Psychological Association, teen stress rivals that of adults, as evidenced by the growing number of kids with anxiety and depression. In fact, young adults today are up to eight times more likely to report symptoms of anxiety and depression than those who lived during the Great Depression.

At the risk of stating the obvious, chronic stress can wreak havoc on health. The Journal of Caring Sciences published a study in 2012 estimating that 35% of American children "experience stress-related health problems." It's no surprise that boys and girls who live with high levels of stress are at a greater risk of everything from obesity to diabetes. And it makes you age faster, as your body is in permanent fight-or-flight.

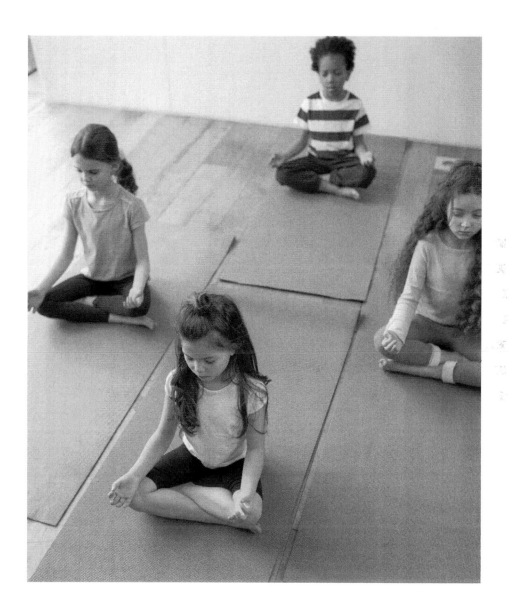

Your child is going to have to deal with stress at some point. It's your job to prepare them to manage stress in a healthy manner

There's no silver bullet for minimizing stress in your children's lives. We have to acknowledge that kids are under an unprecedented amount of stress nowadays. With everything from the influence of social media to growing societal pressure, your child is going to have to deal with stress at some point. It's your job to prepare them to manage stress in a healthy manner. My preferred technique is meditation. I both model the practice to my children and have encouraged them to begin their own. By introducing your children to meditation at a young age, they will have a practice that helps them cope with stress before they actually experience any.

There is a tremendous amount of research outlining the benefits of meditation. To start, it counteracts the aforementioned fight-or-flight response, which in turn reduces the amount of cortisol and adrenaline released. It also can help you control insulin levels, improve heart health, and reduce disorders ranging from insomnia to fibromyalgia. No wonder so many opinion leaders, including Oprah and Beyonce, practice meditation. Oprah even so eloquently described the benefits of meditation when she said: "That way of being 'still' with ourselves – coming back to the center and recognizing that something is more important than you – it's more important than the work you are doing, brings a kind of energy, an intention that we have never had before."

I took my son to meditation classes while we were traveling so he would have a positive, relaxing association with the practice. During the class, we closed our eyes and sat in lotus pose in a beautiful place overlooking a lake. Children as young as four can get meditation training, too. A long list of studies have shown that meditation can reduce not just stress but things like cholesterol and the chance of heart failure.

The best part of meditation, though, is that there's no wrong way to do it. Your children can start with a simple breathing practice, download one of the many apps that teach meditation, or participate in activities that have meditation built in, like walking or listening to music. If you and your children are new to meditation, start with a breathing exercise before bed. Then, gradually increase the amount of time spent meditating. Take them on walks where you set an intention beforehand, use the walk to meditate, then discuss what came up for each other when you get back home. The joy of meditation is that it's a practice that will always be with you. Paul McCartney put it best when he said, "Meditation is a lifelong gift. It's something you can call on at any time."

Many schools are starting to incorporate meditation and mindfulness into their curriculums and after-school activities, too. The Harvard Graduate School of Education even published a study showing that the sixth graders who participated showed "a reduction in perceived stress and modest but significant improvements in sustained attention" and went on to say that further brain imaging showed there was a notable reduced response in the parts of the brain that process stress and negative stimuli. This is great news from a health and longevity perspective. Hopefully, by the time our children are adults, meditating will be as much a part of their daily routines as brushing their teeth.

CHAPTER 9

BE KIND AND GRATEFUL

Let's imagine, for a minute, that your children are already grown. They eat their veggies, get regular exercise, and drink a lot of water. Great! But are they happy? The tough reality is that being healthy doesn't necessarily mean being happy, kind or grateful. That's why it's important for moms and pops to model a good outlook on life—one that includes kindness and gratitude—in addition to modeling other healthy habits.

As parents we have constant reminders of things to be grateful for, as our kids provide us with endless moments where we get to participate in one of the most wonderful aspects of being a human: parenthood. And it's when we step into our gratitude—and truly consider what we have, rather than what we need—that we have the clarity and peace of mind to approach the world with patience and understanding. By practicing gratitude, it makes way for us to be kind, empathetic, considerate people. As the famous Roman statesman and orator Cicero once said, "Gratitude is not only the greatest of virtues, but the parent of all the others."

One time, I was tucking Timothy in when he was around five years old. I asked him what five things he was the most grateful for. I thought he would likely struggle to answer the question, but he immediately listed things: his teacher, his mom, his dog, and so on. Many kids have an embedded sense of gratefulness. They have a beautiful perception of the world—one that we tend to lose when we become adults.

As a parent, you should reinforce gratitude and kindness so your kids will carry those things with them all through life. While it might seem easy enough to just dive into working on this with just your children, I think that it's always a great idea to also adopt a practice on your own. In the beginning, keep it simple and before bed each night, simply speak aloud 3 or 5 things about your day that you were grateful for. This practice will start opening you up to the mindset, and eventually the positive feelings of gratitude will start working their way into your day to day view of the world. And as you're working on gratitude and kindness with your children, you'll also be practicing and living in a way that your kids see and internalize.

But when reinforcing gratitude and kindness with your kids, I think bedtime is the easiest place to start. Building on mindfulness, I recommend having your kids express gratitude then do breathing exercises or meditation before they go to bed each night. You can start simple and have your kids list 3 things they were grateful for, and then do 3 minutes of a breathing exercise or meditation. As it becomes more of a nightly practice, you can up the number and even pair it with the length of your nightly breath exercise.

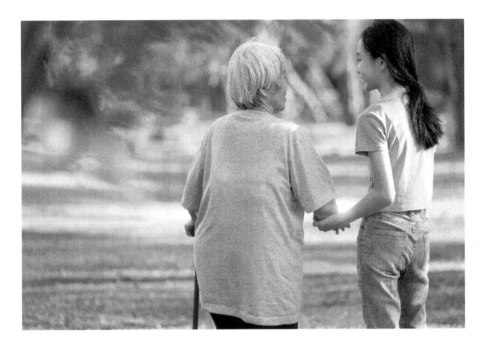

The important part here is repetition and being a reliable positive daily influence on your kids. It takes consistency for gratitude to truly become a habit. But if you and your family stick with it, you'll start looking for things to be thankful for. It's led to a huge change in my overall outlook.

There's a lot of research documenting the link between gratitude and health, too. One study at the Boston University School of Medicine followed over 70,000 individuals for 10 to 30 years. Researchers found that optimism is related to anywhere from an 11% to 15% longer lifespan. By modeling and encouraging gratitude each day, you're instilling important values in your children. They'll appreciate what they have instead of always wanting more.

Gratitude is a personal recognition of the positivity in the world, kindness is the way process of putting gratitude into action and sharing it with the world

It's when you've settled into a solid groove with your daily practice of gratitude, that kindness will also come second nature to you and your kids. As I've alluded to before, gratitude begets kindness. If gratitude is a personal recognition of the positivity in the world, then kindness is the process of putting gratitude into action and sharing it with the world.

Take small opportunities to speak to and about others kindly, to help those in need, and try and find the good in small daily setbacks. Take your kids to volunteer and give back to the community. Participate in charity and teach your kids to do the same. If they get an allowance, tell them to keep 10% and at the end of every year, match the amount they've saved and pick out a charity to donate to together. Instill in your children that by living a good life and being a good person, they can achieve great things and do so in a way that will live on even after they're gone. Like the pop star Taylor Swift once said, "No matter what happens in life, be good to people. Being good to people is a wonderful legacy to leave behind."

Remember—you want your children to have a good quality life, not just a long one.

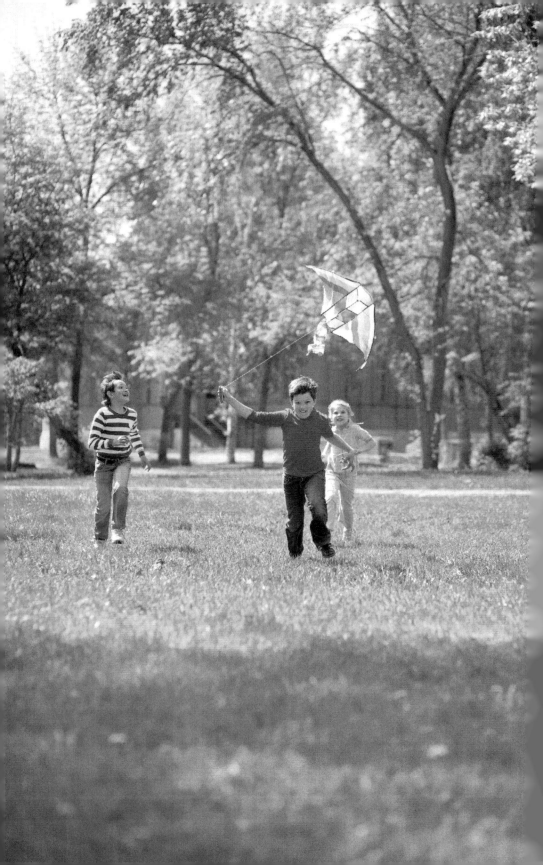

CHAPTER 10

SOCIALIZE!

Another aspect of health that sometimes gets forgotten is the importance of friendships and strong community ties. Put simply, people with larger, more diverse social networks have been shown to live longer. One study of nearly 7,000 adults in California showed that men and women with the fewest social ties were more than twice as likely to die than those with the greatest social ties.

The good news is that most kids are ... well ... kids! They want to go outside and be social, they interact with peers at school, and they're introduced to new people regularly. If your kids are naturally social, make sure to reinforce that behavior. Encourage them to continue finding new friends and talking to new people even when they have already established a circle of besties. This will ensure that they can build new social ties in addition to maintaining established ones.

If your children are a bit more on the shy side, work to build up their confidence. One great strategy is to take whatever activity they love and excel at—whether art, music, sports, etc.—and build their social life around that. A talented young musician is more likely to feel confident and outgoing during a group music lesson, for example. They're in their element, so it's easier to make connections.

Research has shown that social ties enhance mental health, in turn lowering the risk of many of the unhealthy behaviors outlined thus far. Also, playing sports is a great way to get your kids moving and being social—both of which will boost their health. There's no bond quite like the bond of a sports teammate. Many friendships that start on youth sports teams end up lasting a lifetime.

Social interactions aren't just about having fun, though. You should also teach your children the importance of giving back. This relates to the idea of gratitude, but takes it a step further. Helping those in need is a positive thing in and of itself. But it's also been shown to offer numerous health benefits, from lower blood pressure to lower rates of depression.

As is the case with most advice in this book, the best way to teach your children about the importance of social ties is to lead by example. Parents have a key role to play in teaching their kids to be social and educating them on the "rules" of social engagement, explaining a concept of boundaries and norms to help them have more positive experiences with kids and adults and play a positive role within a social set up.

If you as a parent are struggling, rely on your friends and community for help. You shouldn't feel isolated if there is something you can't figure out for yourself. Instead, build relationships, help when you have the opportunity to help, and ask for help when you need it.

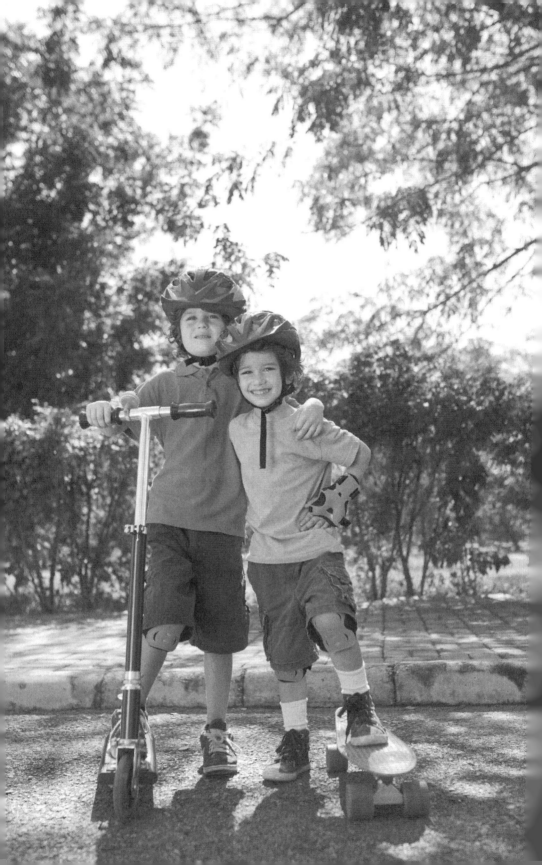

CHAPTER 11

STAY SAFE

Our final component of health and longevity is about using common sense.

Diet, movement, and community are important parts of a healthy lifestyle. But in order to extend your lifespan and those of your children, other risks should be minimized as well. Teach your children that they need to make good choices regarding general safety, which includes everything from safe driving to avoiding drugs and alcohol.

It's pretty easy to forget that our children are essentially walking sponges, just soaking up every situation around them. We are role models for our children in every moment, even during the most mundane activities throughout our day. In fact, these moments often make the largest impression. Tasks like choosing to drive safely, drinking lots of water, or eating healthy can be easy to forget. Still, they are essential to fostering an environment that our children can thrive in now and down the line.

One of many aspects of safety lies in our use of vehicles. Car accidents are the top cause of death for young adults aged 16 to 24. We rarely think that our actions behind the wheel make that much of an impression on our kids, but even things like using our phone while behind the wheel can subtly but seriously influence our children. A recent study conducted by Liberty Mutual concluded that our influence on our children's driving is much more prevalent than one might think. The survey stated that 20% of adults admitted to texting and 37% of adults admitted to using a mobile app while driving. Our influence as parents shows in similar percentages amongst teens: 18% admitted to texting and 38% admitted to using a mobile app while driving. Almost identical percentages.

"Parents are role models for their teen drivers and when the parent is the 'rule breaker' they are setting a bad example," Dr. Gene Beresin, executive director of The Clay Center for Young Healthy Minds at Massachusetts General Hospital said. And keep in mind, this is just what drivers across the board admitted to! One could only imagine the actual numbers. Still, the song remains the same: the kids are always watching!

Once we put the phone down, our job isn't necessarily done. There are many other aspects to how we approach driving that require some attention. Conscientious driving is probably the most basic way to lead by example. Do your best to remain an assertive driver, while refraining from being too aggressive. Simple things like yielding to pedestrians, stopping for yellow lights, and doing your best to remain patient and calm in otherwise stressful situations, are easy ways to positively reinforce healthy, safe driving habits for your future drivers.

One of the largest and most obvious things to consider is the relationship we show our kids between alcohol and driving. And by this I mean there should be no relationship between alcohol and driving. This means never drinking and then getting behind the wheel. As a parent, always take a taxi or public transit if you've consumed alcohol. And don't be afraid to have an open conversation with your kids if you find yourself in a situation where you've consumed alcohol and the choice to drive home presents itself. I think it's okay to announce that you're choosing to take an Uber or Lyft home because you've had something to drink. In doing so, it brings up the topic of drinking and driving, and provides your children with a safe option they can recall later in life if they ever find themselves in a similar situation.

This approach also allows parents to remove some possible stigma around drinking by showing kids they can have a healthy relationship with alcohol while remaining responsible and considerate. Once again, children learn a lot by simply watching you. Take the opportunities to move situations into actual discussions, rather than relying on the unspoken game of "monkey see, monkey do."

As your kids grow up, be sure to teach them about the dangers of drugs and alcohol as well. Unfortunately, there's been an uptick in opioid and alcohol abuse in the United States—to the point that overall life expectancy in the U.S. is actually on the decline. Specifically looking at opioids, some unfortunate statistics have come to light regarding children's exposure to them in recent years. According to a study released in the Official Journal of the American Academy of Pediatrics, "From 2006 to 2012, [more than] 22,000 children were treated in US emergency departments for opioid poisoning."

The study goes on to say that these exposures to prescription opioids during childhood, often leads to future use of illegal substances: "almost 80% of new heroin users have previously used opioid pain medications." While this is deeply upsetting to learn, it forces us to reconcile with the truth: at some point, your children will be exposed to people who drink and use drugs, whether accidentally or intentionally. Begin having conversations about these substances early so they're prepared to make healthy decisions when the situation arises.

Finally, while I've praised sports as an opportunity for physical fitness and building social ties, it's important to remember that some sports are riskier than others. About 10% of traumatic brain injuries happen during sports, with football and basketball causing the most head injuries for children under 14. Be aware of these risks as you sign your children up for sports and keep a close eye out for injuries.

Sergey Young

10 LONGEVITY TIPS FOR KIDS

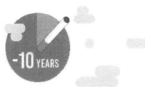

-10 YEARS

1 DON'T SMOKE

Instill in your kids the knowledge that smoking or doing drugs is dangerous

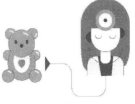

2 DRINK WATER

Avoid sugary drinks to set a good example to your kids and teach them to drink more water

3 BEFRIEND A DOCTOR

Take your kids to a family doctor on a regular basis for check-ups

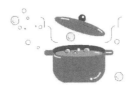

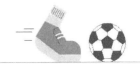

4 LEARN TO COOK HEALTHY

Feed your kids plant-based meals and organic meat and poultry. Teach them to cook their own food and why homemade meals are healthier than fast and processed foods

5 MOVE DAILY

Accustom your kids to regular physical activity, teach them different types of exercises: yoga, cardio and resistance training. Bond with your kids on daily walks and regular hikes

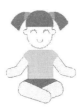

6 LIMIT USE OF GADGETS

Limit entertainment use of technological gadgets to 20 min per day. Encourage kids to read paper books

7 MEDITATE

Introduce your kids to meditation techniques and encourage them to get into the habit of doing it every day. Start with a simple breathing meditation

8 BE KIND AND GRATEFUL

Teach your kids the importance of being kind to others and grateful for what they have

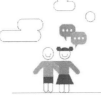

SAFETY FIRST

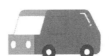

9 BE SOCIAL

Help your kids to discover the value of friendship and community support

10 STAY SAFE

Explain to your kids the importance of making good choices regarding general safety: responsible driving, hygiene, social distancing when needed. And no extreme sports, please :)

Connect with me on:

Website:
sergeyyoung.com

Facebook:
sergeyyoung200

Linkedin:
Sergey You

CONCLUSION

Parenting is one of the most challenging and most rewarding roles most adults experience in their lifetimes. My four kids are the joy of my life. I've learned so much from them. Hopefully, they've learned from me too. Mothers and fathers naturally want to keep their kids safe, happy, and healthy. But in order to do so, we must think long-term. The goal is to set boys and girls up for health and longevity, which refers to both how long our kids will live and what kind of quality their lives will have.

In this book, we went through ten areas that I think are most important for teaching boys and girls lasting, healthy habits.

We started with the importance of teaching kids to make healthy and educated food choices, that they will exercise even outside of the household, by shopping and cooking together, growing simple herbs on a balcony, or visiting a local farm. We learned how eliminating unhealthy foods, snacks, and drinks from your kitchen and packing whole, unprocessed lunch to school could play a key role in the process of adopting a healthy eating mindset!

We looked at the next piece of the good health and longevity puzzle: the value of staying hydrated and choosing water over sugary and caffeinated drinks. And how you can help your kids fall in love with water by making it fun: adding berries, lemon or mint leaves in the water or letting them pick a water bottle with a favorite cartoon character!

We discussed how befriending a family doctor and scheduling a regular visit to his office could help your kids avoid life-threatening diseases in the future and stay up to date with all the development the future healthcare will have to offer!

We explored how exercise and a habit of being active daily, even without practicing sport, could help your kids minimize the risk of physical and mental health problems. And how you can help them get accustomed to active life by setting an example despite being a busy parent.

We dug into the importance of sleep, how we can make sure our kids get enough Zzzs per night and they are as restorative and rejuvenating as possible.

We had a close look at how uncontrolled use of gadgets can affect health and potentially longevity and the wise way to manage your kids' screen time.

We reviewed how a simple meditation routine could help reduce stress and anxiety in our kids' lives and help them grow stronger and healthier.

We talked about aspects that often get forgotten in the longevity discourse--the power of kindness, gratitude, and being social, the link they have with health and lifespans, and how parents can reinforce these qualities in their kids.

Lastly, we emphasized the significance of common sense in our day-to-day choices. Avoiding drugs and alcohol, especially when driving, following safety rules inside a vehicle: no cell phones while driving, no speeding, and always using safety belts minimize risks of accidents that can shorten our lives. Here and in all discussed aspects, we, parents, have a critical role by setting up a good example!

The 10 habits for raising healthy kids are simple concepts that will enhance the quality and quantity of your kids' lives—especially if they're done in a fun manner! I outlined these principles in a simple infographic that you

Download infographic here: sergeyyoung.com/10-longevity-tips-for-kids

can download at https://sergeyyoung.com/10-longevity-tips-for-kids, print it out and stick to your fridge.

The earlier you can start your children on a healthy path, the better. There will be fewer bad habits for them to unlearn, fewer health problems for them to overcome, and more years of health and happiness for them to enjoy.

But I hope that you've taken this information, and let it excite you to the possibilities you're capable of exploring with parenting. We not only want what's best for our children, but in many ways, we want them to be better people than we are.

It's my sincere hope that these ten areas help you in your journey towards raising healthy, happy and successful children.

What more could a parent ask for?

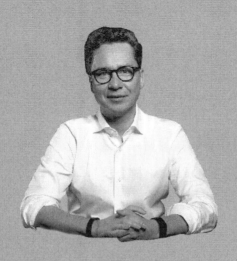

WANT TO KNOW MORE?

SIGN UP TO MY NEWSLETTER:

SergeyYoung.com/newsletter

AND CONNECT WITH ME
ON SOCIAL MEDIA

Facebook.com/**SergeyYoung200**

Linkedin.com/in/**SergeyYoung**

Instagram.com/**SergeyYoung200**

REFERENCES

CHAPTER 1: Introduction

Centers for Disease Control and Prevention. «Life Expectancy»

https://www.cdc.gov/nchs/fastats/life-expectancy.htm

Census. «Aging population»

https://www.census.gov/newsroom/releases/archives/aging_population/cb11-194.html#:~:text=The%20nation's%2090%2Dand%2Dolder,projected%20to%20more%20than%20quadruple.

Chapter 2: You are what you eat

TuftsNow. May 30, 2021. «National study finds diets remain poor for most American children; disparities persist»

https://now.tufts.edu/news-releases/national-study-finds-diets-remain-poor-most-american-children-disparities-persist

The New York Times. March 17, 2005. «Children's Life Expectancy Being Cut Short by Obesity»

https://www.nytimes.com/2005/03/17/health/childrens-life-expectancy-being-cut-short-by-obesity.html

Health.gov. President's Council on Sports, Fitness & Nutrition.

https://www.hhs.gov/fitness/resource-center/facts-and-statistics/index.html#footnote-13

National Library of Medicine. August 27, 2011. «Health and economic burden of the projected obesity trends in the USA and the UK»

https://pubmed.ncbi.nlm.nih.gov/21872750/

Moms. October 22, 2018. «How These 20 Celebs Are Feeding Their Kids»

https://www.moms.com/how-these-20-celebs-are-feeding-their-kids/

Bright Side. «17 Strict Rules Taken Right Out of Celebrity Parenting

Books»

https://brightside.me/wonder-people/17-strict-rules-taken-right-out-of-celebrity-parenting-books-510460

CNN Health. May 17, 2019. «Overprocessed foods add 500 calories to your diet every day, causing weight gain»

https://edition.cnn.com/2019/05/17/health/ultraprocessed-foods-weight-gain-study-trnd/index.html

Time. August 1, 2019. «Is Sugar as Bad for Kids as It Is for Adults?»

https://time.com/5640428/sugar-kids-vs-adults/

Chapter 3: Fall in love with water!

US National Library of Medicine. January 10, 2018 «Sources of Added Sugars in Young Children, Adolescents, and Adults with Low and High Intakes of Added Sugars»

https://www.ncbi.nlm.nih.gov/pmc/articles/PMC5793330/

Cleveland Clinic. January 4, 2018. «Sugar: How Bad Are Sweets for Your Kids?»

https://health.clevelandclinic.org/sugar-how-bad-are-sweets-for-your-kids/

The New York Times. March 21, 2019. «Sugary Drinks Tied To Shorter Lifespan»

https://www.nytimes.com/2019/03/21/well/eat/sugary-drinks-tied-to-shorter-life-span.html

National Library of Medicine. «Substituting sugar-sweetened beverages with water or milk is inversely associated with body fatness development from childhood to adolescence»

https://pubmed.ncbi.nlm.nih.gov/25441586/

Kids Health from Nemours. «Why Drinking Water Is the Way to Go»

https://kidshealth.org/en/kids/water.html#:~:text=Without%20oxygen%2C%20those%20tiny%20cells,and%20get%20rid%20of%20waste

HealthyChildren.ogr. «Choose Water for Healthy Hydration»

https://www.healthychildren.org/English/healthy-living/nutrition/Pages/Choose-Water-for-Healthy-Hydration.aspx

Chapter 4: Befriend your doctor

Freenome https://www.freenome.com/

Exo Imaging https://www.exo.inc/

Eko Health https://www.ekohealth.com/

Cardiology 2.0. September 24, 2019. «Cardiac MRI Scans Analysis in just 4 seconds; AI makes it Faster and Precise»

https://cardiology2.com/cardiac-mri-scans-analysis-in-just-4-seconds-ai-makes-it-faster-and-precise/

Chapter 5: Get movin'!

Science Direct. November 28, 1953. «Coronary Heart-Disease and Physical Activity of Work»

https://www.sciencedirect.com/science/article/abs/pii/S0140673653914950

Brigham and Women's Hospital and

Harvard Medical School, Harvard School of Public Health, Boston, MA. «Physical activity and all-cause mortality: what is the dose-response relation?»

http://citeseerx.ist.psu.edu/viewdoc/download?doi=10.1.1.460.957&rep=rep1&type=pdf

Wiley Online Library. «Major public health benefits of physical activity»

https://onlinelibrary.wiley.com/doi/full/10.1002/art.10907

Cancer Trends Progress Report.

https://progressreport.cancer.gov/sites/default/files/archive/report2019.pdf

Live Science. «Exercise Boosts Life Expectancy, Study Finds»

https://www.livescience.com/36723-exercise-life-expectancy-overweight-obese.html

Health.gov. «2008 Physical Activity Guidelines for Americans»

https://health.gov/our-work/physical-activity/previous-guidelines/2008-physical-activity-guidelines

Stanford Children's Health. «Organized sports for kids»

https://www.stanfordchildrens.org/en/topic/default?id=organized-sports-for-kids-1-4556

Jama Network. «Association of Participation in Team Sports With Depression, Current Depressive Symptoms, and Anxiety Among Males and Females»

https://jamanetwork.com/journals/jamapediatrics/fullarticle/2734743

Harvard Health Publishing. April 19, 2021. «Walking: Your steps to health»

https://www.health.harvard.edu/staying-healthy/walking-your-steps-to-health

Science Direct. January 2003. «Adolescent participation in sports and adult physical activity»

https://www.sciencedirect.com/science/article/abs/pii/S0749379702005755?casa_token=rRQEWIYt_WoAAAAA:grIESU1jLA0Po3Sz4DsHxp-FSdLGnvhAr-uUrf_RTtOcBaUj7wYWZWQeDggT6zps94nVcXZBH48

Chapter 6: Prioritize rest

Centers for Disease Control and Prevention. «Data and Statistics.

Short Sleep Duration Among US Adults»

https://www.cdc.gov/sleep/data_statistics.html

Sleep Foundation. September 24, 2020. Children and sleep.

https://www.sleepfoundation.org/children-and-sleep

Sleep Foundation. October 23, 2020. «What is White Noise?»

https://www.sleepfoundation.org/bedroom-environment/white-noise

Chapter 7: Use gadgets wisely

World Health Organization. April 24, 2019. «To grow up healthy, children need to sit less and play more»

https://www.who.int/news/item/24-04-2019-to-grow-up-healthy-children-need-to-sit-less-and-play-more

Centers for Disease Control and Prevention. Screen Time vs. Lean Time Infographic.

https://www.cdc.gov/nccdphp/dnpao/

multimedia/infographics/getmoving.
html#:~:text=According%20to%20the
%20Kaiser%20Family,watching%20a%
20screen%20for%20fun

Jama Network. January 28, 2019.
«Association Between Screen Time
and Children's Performance on a
Developmental Screening Test»

https://jamanetwork.com/journals/ja
mapediatrics/fullarticle/2722666

Official Journal of the American
Academy of Pediatrics. November
2007.

«Digital Media and Sleep in Childhood
and Adolescence»

https://pediatrics.aappublications.org/
content/140/Supplement_2/S92

BMJ Journal. «Screen time is
associated with adiposity and insulin
resistance in children»

https://adc.bmj.com/content/102/7/612

HealthyChildren.ogr. «AAP
Announces New Recommendations
for Children's Media Use»

https://www.healthychildren.org/Engli
sh/news/Pages/AAP-Announces-
New-Recommendations-for-
Childrens-Media-Use.aspx

Huffpost. 7 July, 2015. «Celebrity
Parents Make Good Screen Sense A
Priority».

https://www.huffpost.com/entry/celeb
rity-screen-
sense_n_559bff08e4b0759e2b510494

Business Insider. «Chrissy Teigen,
master of the Twitter clapback and
author of the cookbook 'Cravings,'
told Harper's Bazaar that she and
husband John Legend 'are not those
people that are like 'no screen time!'»

https://www.businessinsider.com/tec
h-free-celebrities-children-family-
screen-time-2019-12#chrissy-teigen-

master-of-the-twitter-clapback-and-
author-of-the-cookbook-cravings-
told-harpers-bazaar-that-she-and-
husband-john-legend-are-not-those-
people-that-are-like-no-screen-time-3

Very Well Family. May 25, 2021. «Best
Educational Apps for Kids»

https://www.verywellfamily.com/best-
educational-apps-for-kids-4842950

Chapter 8: Teach meditation

NCBI. «Stress and Health:
Psychological, Behavioral, and
Biological Determinants»

https://www.ncbi.nlm.nih.gov/pmc/art
icles/PMC2568977/

Wtop News. «More kids plagued with
chronic stress: Why it's happening,
how to help»

https://wtop.com/parenting/2018/02/
more-kids-plagued-with-chronic-
stress-why-its-happening-how-to-
help/

NCBI. «Investigation of Stress
Symptoms among Primary School
Children»

https://www.ncbi.nlm.nih.gov/pmc/art
icles/PMC4166684/

Center for Anxiety Disorders. «How
Stress Affects Child Development»

https://centerforanxietydisorders.com
/stress-affects-child-
development/#:~:text=The%20inciden
ce%20of%20obesity%2C%20diabetes,
and%20domestic%20violence%20gre
atly%20increase

International Journal of Yoga. 2018.
«Effect of 6 months of meditation on
blood sugar, glycosylated
hemoglobin, and insulin levels in
patients of coronary artery disease»

https://www.ijoy.org.in/article.asp?issn=0973-6131;year=2018;volume=11;issue=2;spage=122;epage=128;aulast=Sinha

Harvard Graduate School of Education. «Mindfulness in the Classroom: Learning from a School-based Mindfulness Intervention through the Boston Charter Research Collaborative»

https://transformingeducation.org/wp-content/uploads/2019/01/2019-BCRC-Mindfulness-Brief.pdf

Chapter 9: Be kind and grateful

Science Daily. «New evidence that optimists live longer»

https://www.sciencedaily.com/releases/2019/08/190826150700.htm

Chapter 10: Socialize!

News in Health. «Do Social Ties Affect Our Health? Exploring the Biology of Relationships»

https://newsinhealth.nih.gov/2017/02/do-social-ties-affect-our-health

American Journal of Epidemiology. February 1, 1979. «Social Networks, Host Resistance, and Mortality: a Nine-Year Follow-Up Study of Alameda County Residents»

https://academic.oup.com/aje/article-abstract/109/2/186/74197

Annual Reviews. «Emotions, Morbidity, and Mortality: New Perspectives from Psychoneuroimmunology»

https://www.annualreviews.org/doi/ab s/10.1146/annurev.psych.53.100901.135217?journalCode=psych&casa_token=2nxypeCel_EAAAAA%3AiLgMUvQ5GefHvMYrTMDIKreZaun4wbC8tSpKdw8gA2aQotkm0VXc5wV4A0IPwQFZCudpETuKb2oztw

Cleveland Clinic. Health Essential. October 28, 2020. «Why Giving Is Good for Your Health»

https://health.clevelandclinic.org/why-giving-is-good-for-your-health/

Chapter 11: Stay safe

Safety Insurance.

https://www.safetyinsurance.com/driversafety/tips_statistics.html

Stat News. February 18, 2021. «U.S. life expectancy fell by a year in the first half of 2020, CDC report finds»

https://www.statnews.com/2021/02/18/u-s-life-expectancy-fell-by-a-year-in-the-first-half-of-2020-cdc-report-finds/#:~:text=Life%20expectancy%20at%20birth%20for,for%20January%20through%20June%202020.

Official Journal of the American Academy of Pediatrics. «Prescription Opioid Exposures Among Children and Adolescents in the United States: 2000–2015»

https://pediatrics.aappublications.org/content/139/4/e20163382

American Association of Neurological Surgeons. «Sports-related Head Injury»

https://www.aans.org/Patients/Neurosurgical-Conditions-and-Treatments/Sports-related-Head-Injury#:~:text=There%20are%20an%20estimated%201.7,to%20sports%20and%20recreational%20activities.

Printed in Great Britain
by Amazon

67639957R00052